Cram101 Textbook Outlines to accompany:

PeriAnesthesia Nursing: A Critical Care Approach

Cecil B. Drain PhD RN CRNA FAAN FASAHP, 5th Edition

A Content Technologies Inc. publication (c) 2012.

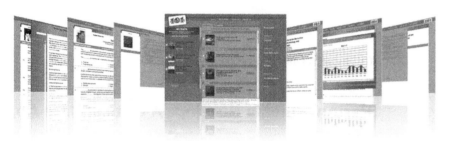

Learning System

Cram101 Textbook Outlines is a learning system. The notes in this book are the highlights of your textbook, you will never have to highlight a book again.

How to use this book. Take this book to class, it is your notebook for the lecture. The notes and highlights on the left hand side of the pages follow the outline and order of the textbook. All you have to do is follow along while your instructor presents the lecture. Circle the items emphasized in class and add other important information on the right side. With Cram101 Textbook Outlines you'll spend less time writing and more time listening. Learning becomes more efficient.

Cram101.com Online

Increase your studying efficiency by using Cram101.com's practice tests and online reference material. It is the perfect complement to Cram101 Textbook Outlines. Use self-teaching matching tests or simulate in-class testing with comprehensive multiple choice tests, or simply use Cram's true and false tests for quick review. Cram101.com even allows you to enter your in-class notes for an integrated studying format combining the textbook notes with your class notes.

Visit **www.Cram101.com**, click Sign Up at the top of the screen, and enter **DK73DW14499** in the promo code box on the registration screen. Your access to www.Cram101.com is discounted by 50% because you have purchased this book. Sign up and stop highlighting textbooks forever.

PeriAnesthesia Nursing: A Critical Care Approach
Cecil B. Drain PhD RN CRNA FAAN FASAHP, 5th

CONTENTS

Chapter 1. Part I The Postanesthesia Care Unit

Antibacterial	An antibacterial is a compound or substance that kills or slows down the growth of bacteria. The term is often used synonymously with the term antibiotic(s); today, however, with increased knowledge of the causative agents of various infectious diseases, antibiotic(s) has come to denote a broader range of antimicrobial compounds, including anti-fungal and other compounds.
Infection control	Infection control is the discipline concerned with preventing nosocomial or healthcare-associated infection. As such, it is a practical (rather than an academic) sub-discipline of epidemiology. It is an essential (though often under-recognized and under-supported) part of the infrastructure of health care.
Cleft lip and palate	Cleft lip (cheiloschisis) and cleft palate (palatoschisis), which can also occur together as cleft lip and palate, are variations of a type of clefting congenital deformity caused by abnormal facial development during gestation. A cleft is a fissure or opening--a gap. It is the non-fusion of the body's natural structures that form before birth.
Pulmonary arteries	The pulmonary arteries carry blood from the heart to the lungs. They are the only arteries (other than umbilical arteries in the fetus) that carry deoxygenated blood.
	In the human heart, the pulmonary trunk begins at the base of the right ventricle.
Malignant hyperthermia	Malignant hyperthermia or malignant hyperpyrexia is a rare life-threatening condition that is usually triggered by exposure to certain drugs used for general anesthesia; specifically, the volatile anesthetic agents and the neuromuscular blocking agent, succinylcholine. In susceptible individuals, these drugs can induce a drastic and uncontrolled increase in skeletal muscle oxidative metabolism, which overwhelms the body's capacity to supply oxygen, remove carbon dioxide, and regulate body temperature, eventually leading to circulatory collapse and death if not treated quickly.
	Susceptibility to Malignant hyperthermia is often inherited as an autosomal dominant disorder, for which there are at least 6 genetic loci of interest, most prominently the ryanodine receptor gene (RYR1).

Clam101

Chapter 1. Part I The Postanesthesia Care Unit

Pain management	Pain management is a branch of medicine employing an interdisciplinary approach for easing the suffering and improving the quality of life of those living with pain. The typical pain management team includes medical practitioners, clinical psychologists, physiotherapists, occupational therapists, and nurse practitioners. Pain sometimes resolves promptly once the underlying trauma or pathology has healed, and is treated by one practitioner, with drugs such as analgesics and (occasionally) anxiolytics.
Receptor antagonist	A Receptor antagonist is a type of receptor ligand or drug that does not provoke a biological response itself upon binding to a receptor, but blocks or dampens agonist-mediated responses. In pharmacology, antagonists have affinity but no efficacy for their cognate receptors, and binding will disrupt the interaction and inhibit the function of an agonist or inverse agonist at receptors. Antagonists mediate their effects by binding to the active site or to allosteric sites on receptors, or they may interact at unique binding sites not normally involved in the biological regulation of the receptor's activity.
Antimicrobial prophylaxis	Antimicrobial prophylaxis refers to the prevention of infection complications using antimicrobial therapy (most commonly antibiotics). Even when sterile techniques are adhered to, surgical procedures can introduce bacteria and other microbes in the blood (causing bacteremia), which can colonize and infect different parts of the body. An estimated 5 to 10 percent of hospitalized patients undergoing otolaryngology ("head and neck") surgery acquire a nosocomial ("hospital") infection, which adds a substantial cost and an average of 4 extra days to the hospital stay.
Aseptic technique	Aseptic technique refers to a procedure that is performed under sterile conditions. This includes medical and laboratory techniques, such as with microbiological cultures. It includes techniques like flame sterilization.
Pathogen	A pathogen is a biological agent such as a virus, bacteria, prion, or fungus that causes disease to its host. There are several substrates including pathways whereby pathogens can invade a host; the principal pathways have different episodic time frames, but soil contamination has the longest or most persistent potential for harboring a pathogen.

CYam101

The body contains many natural orders of defense against some of the common pathogens (such as Pneumocystis) in the form of the human immune system and by some "helpful" bacteria present in the human body's normal flora.

Transmission

In medicine, transmission is the passing of a disease from an infected individual or group to a previously uninfected individual or group. The microorganisms (bacteria and viruses) that cause disease may be transmitted from one person to another by one or more of the following means:

· droplet contact - coughing or sneezing on another person

· direct physical contact - touching an infected person, including sexual contact

· indirect contact - usually by touching soil contamination or a contaminated surface

· airborne transmission - if the microorganism can remain in the air for long periods

· fecal-oral transmission - usually from contaminated food or water sources

· vector borne transmission - carried by insects or other animals

Microorganisms vary widely in the length of time that they can survive outside the human body, and so vary in how they are transmitted.

Disease can be transmitted in two ways:

· Horizontal disease transmission - from one individual to another in the same generation (peers in the same age group). Horizontal transmission can occur by either direct contact (licking, touching, biting), or indirect contact .

Chapter 1. Part I The Postanesthesia Care Unit

	· Vertical disease transmission - passing a disease causing agent vertically from parent to offspring. Typically the mother transmits the disease by means of bodily fluid, and sometimes breast milk.
Microorganism	A Microorganism or microbe is an organism that is microscopic . The study of Microorganisms is called microbiology, a subject that began with Anton van Leeuwenhoek's discovery of Microorganisms in 1675, using a microscope of his own design. Microorganisms are very diverse; they include bacteria, fungi, archaea, and protists; microscopic plants (green algae); and animals such as plankton and the planarian.
Myringotomy	Myringotomy is a surgical procedure in which a tiny incision is created in the eardrum, so as to relieve pressure caused by the excessive build-up of fluid, or to drain pus. Myringotomy is often performed as a treatment for otitis media. If a patient requires myringotomy for drainage or ventilation of the middle ear, this generally implies that the Eustachian tube is either partially or completely obstructed and is not able to perform this function in its usual physiologic fashion.
Patient education	Patient education is the process by which health professionals and others impart information to patients that will alter their health behaviors or improve their health status. Education providers may include: physicians, registered dietitians, nurses, hospital discharge planners, medical social workers, psychologists, disease or disability advocacy groups, special interest groups, and pharmaceutical companies.
Local anesthetic	A local anesthetic is a drug that causes reversible local anesthesia and a loss of nociception. When it is used on specific nerve pathways (nerve block), effects such as analgesia (loss of pain sensation) and paralysis (loss of muscle power) can be achieved. Clinical local anesthetics belong to one of two classes: aminoamide and aminoester local anesthetics.
Anesthesia	Anesthesia, traditionally meant the condition of having sensation (including the feeling of pain) blocked or temporarily taken away. It is a pharmacologically induced and reversible state of amnesia, analgesia, loss of responsiveness, loss of skeletal muscle reflexes or decreased stress response, or all simultaneously. This allows patients to undergo surgery and other procedures without the distress and pain they would otherwise experience.

Chapter 1. Part I The Postanesthesia Care Unit

Thrombosis	Thrombosis is the formation of a blood clot inside a blood vessel, obstructing the flow of blood through the circulatory system. When a blood vessel is injured, the body uses platelets and fibrin to form a blood clot to prevent blood loss. If the clotting is too severe and the clot breaks free, the traveling clot is now know as an embolus.
Tracheal intubation	Tracheal intubation, usually simply referred to as intubation, is the placement of a flexible plastic tube into the trachea (windpipe) to maintain an open airway or to serve as a conduit through which to administer certain drugs. It is frequently performed in critically injured, ill or anesthetized patients to facilitate ventilation of the lungs, including mechanical ventilation, and to prevent the possibility of asphyxiation or airway obstruction. The most widely used route is orotracheal, in which an endotracheal tube is passed through the mouth and vocal apparatus into the trachea.

Chapter 2. Part II Physiologig Considerations in the PACU

Anesthesia	Anesthesia, traditionally meant the condition of having sensation (including the feeling of pain) blocked or temporarily taken away. It is a pharmacologically induced and reversible state of amnesia, analgesia, loss of responsiveness, loss of skeletal muscle reflexes or decreased stress response, or all simultaneously. This allows patients to undergo surgery and other procedures without the distress and pain they would otherwise experience.
Receptor antagonist	A Receptor antagonist is a type of receptor ligand or drug that does not provoke a biological response itself upon binding to a receptor, but blocks or dampens agonist-mediated responses. In pharmacology, antagonists have affinity but no efficacy for their cognate receptors, and binding will disrupt the interaction and inhibit the function of an agonist or inverse agonist at receptors. Antagonists mediate their effects by binding to the active site or to allosteric sites on receptors, or they may interact at unique binding sites not normally involved in the biological regulation of the receptor`s activity.
Local anesthetic	A local anesthetic is a drug that causes reversible local anesthesia and a loss of nociception. When it is used on specific nerve pathways (nerve block), effects such as analgesia (loss of pain sensation) and paralysis (loss of muscle power) can be achieved. Clinical local anesthetics belong to one of two classes: aminoamide and aminoester local anesthetics.
Defibrillation	Defibrillation is the definitive treatment for the life-threatening cardiac arrhythmias, ventricular fibrillation and pulseless ventricular tachycardia. Defibrillation consists of delivering a therapeutic dose of electrical energy to the affected heart with a device called a defibrillator. This depolarizes a critical mass of the heart muscle, terminates the arrhythmia, and allows normal sinus rhythm to be reestablished by the body's natural pacemaker, in the sinoatrial node of the heart.
Hypovolemia	In physiology and medicine, Hypovolemia is a state of decreased blood volume; more specifically, decrease in volume of blood plasma. It is thus the intravascular component of volume contraction (or loss of blood volume due to things such as hemorrhaging or dehydration), but, as it also is the most essential one, Hypovolemia and volume contraction are sometimes used synonymously. It differs from dehydration, which is defined as excessive loss of body water.

Chapter 2. Part II Physiologig Considerations in the PACU

Lidocaine	Lidocaine (Xylocaine) or lignocaine (/ˈlɪ?gn?keɪ?n/) (former BAN) is a common local anesthetic and antiarrhythmic drug. Lidocaine is used topically to relieve itching, burning and pain from skin inflammations, injected as a dental anesthetic or as a local anesthetic for minor surgery.
	History
	Lidocaine, the first amino amide-type local anesthetic, was first synthesized under the name Xylocaine by Swedish chemist Nils Löfgren in 1943. His colleague Bengt Lundqvist performed the first injection anesthesia experiments on himself.
Ptosis	Ptosis is a (drooping) of the upper or lower eyelid. The drooping may be worse after being awake longer, when the individual's muscles are tired. This condition is sometimes called "lazy eye", but that term normally refers to amblyopia.
Transmission	In medicine, transmission is the passing of a disease from an infected individual or group to a previously uninfected individual or group. The microorganisms (bacteria and viruses) that cause disease may be transmitted from one person to another by one or more of the following means:
	· droplet contact - coughing or sneezing on another person
	· direct physical contact - touching an infected person, including sexual contact
	· indirect contact - usually by touching soil contamination or a contaminated surface
	· airborne transmission - if the microorganism can remain in the air for long periods
	· fecal-oral transmission - usually from contaminated food or water sources
	· vector borne transmission - carried by insects or other animals
	Microorganisms vary widely in the length of time that they can survive outside the human body, and so vary in how they are transmitted.

Disease can be transmitted in two ways:

· Horizontal disease transmission - from one individual to another in the same generation (peers in the same age group). Horizontal transmission can occur by either direct contact (licking, touching, biting), or indirect contact .

· Vertical disease transmission - passing a disease causing agent vertically from parent to offspring. Typically the mother transmits the disease by means of bodily fluid, and sometimes breast milk.

Topical anesthetic	A topical anesthetic is a local anesthetic that is used to numb the surface of a body part. They can be used to numb any area of the skin as well as the front of the eyeball, the inside of the nose, ear or throat, the anus and the genital area. Topical anesthetics are available in creams, ointments, aerosols, sprays, lotions, and jellies.
Hypoventilation	In medicine, Hypoventilation occurs when ventilation is inadequate (hypo means 'below') to perform needed gas exchange. By definition it causes an increased concentration of carbon dioxide (hypercapnia) and respiratory acidosis. It can be caused by medical conditions, such as stroke affecting the brainstem, by holding one's breath, or by drugs, typically when taken in overdose.
Methemoglobin	Methemoglobin is a form of the oxygen-carrying protein hemoglobin , in which the iron in the heme group is in the Fe^{3+} (ferric) state, not the Fe^{2+} (ferrous) of normal hemoglobin. Methemoglobin cannot carry oxygen. It is a bluish chocolate-brown in color.
Airway	The pulmonary Airway comprises those parts of the respiratory system through which air flows, conceptually beginning (on inhalation from the external environment) at the nose and mouth, and terminating in the alveoli. It is generally used synonymously with respiratory tract, to avoid sounding overly scientific. From the mouth or nose, inhaled air passes through the pharynx into the trachea, where it separates into the left and right main bronchi at the carina, situated at the level of the second thoracic vertebra.

Chapter 2. Part II Physiologig Considerations in the PACU

Dead space	In physiology, dead space is air that is inhaled by the body in breathing, but does not take part in gas exchange. Not all the air in each breath is able to be used for the exchange of oxygen and carbon dioxide. About a third of every resting breath is exhaled exactly as it came into the body.
Oropharynx	The Oropharynx reaches from the Uvula to the level of the hyoid bone.
	It opens anteriorly, through the isthmus faucium, into the mouth, while in its lateral wall, between the two palatine arches, is the palatine tonsil.
	Although older resources have stated that Fusobacterium is a common occurrence in the human Oropharynx, the current consensus is that Fusobacterium should always be treated as a pathogen.
	The name is formed from their initials:
	· Haemophilus
	· Actinobacillus actinomycetemcomitans
	· Cardiobacterium hominis
	· Eikenella corrodens
	· Kingella
	All of these organisms are part of the normal oropharyngeal flora which grow slowly, prefer a carbon dioxide-enriched atmosphere and share an enhanced capacity to produce endocardial infections, especially in young children.

Chapter 2. Part II Physiologig Considerations in the PACU

Laryngospasm	In medicine, laryngospasm is an uncontrolled/involuntary muscular contraction (spasm) of the laryngeal cords. The condition typically lasts less than 60 seconds, and causes a partial blocking of breathing in, while breathing out remains easier. It may be triggered when the vocal cords or the area of the trachea below the cords detects the entry of water, mucus, blood, or other substance.
Recurrent laryngeal nerve	The Recurrent laryngeal nerve is a branch of the vagus nerve (tenth cranial nerve) that supplies motor function and sensation to the larynx (voice box). It travels within the endoneurial sheath. It is the nerve of the 6th Branchial Arch.
Pulse oximetry	Pulse oximetry is a non-invasive method allowing the monitoring of the oxygenation of a patient's hemoglobin. A sensor is placed on a thin part of the patient's body, usually a fingertip or earlobe, or in the case of a neonate, across a foot, and a light containing both red and infrared wavelengths is passed from one side to the other. Changing absorbance of each of the two wavelengths is measured, allowing determination of the absorbances due to the pulsing arterial blood alone, excluding venous blood, skin, bone, muscle, fat, and (in most cases) fingernail polish.
Sensor	A Sensor is a device that measures a physical quantity and converts it into a signal which can be read by an observer or by an instrument. For example, a mercury-in-glass thermometer converts the measured temperature into expansion and contraction of a liquid which can be read on a calibrated glass tube. A thermocouple converts temperature to an output voltage which can be read by a voltmeter.
Upper respiratory tract	The upper respiratory tract primarily refers to the parts of the respiratory system lying outside of the thorax or above the sternal angle. Another definition commomly used in medicine is the airway above the glottis or vocal cords. Some specify that the glottis (vocal cords) is the defining line between the upper and lower respiratory tracts; yet even others make the line at the cricoid cartilage.
Pulmonary edema	Pulmonary edema is fluid accumulation in the lungs. It leads to impaired gas exchange and may cause respiratory failure. It is due to either failure of the heart to remove fluid from the lung circulation or a direct injury to the lung parenchyma .

Chapter 2. Part II Physiologig Considerations in the PACU

Ventricular assist device	A Ventricular assist device, is a mechanical circulatory device that is used to partially or completely replace the function of a failing heart. Some Ventricular assist devices are intended for short term use, typically for patients recovering from heart attacks or heart surgery, while others are intended for long term use (months to years and in some cases for life), typically for patients suffering from congestive heart failure. Ventricular assist devices need to be clearly distinguished from artificial hearts, which are designed to completely take over cardiac function and generally require the removal of the patient's heart.
Chloroprocaine	Chloroprocaine (often in the hydrochloride salt form as the aforementioned trade names) is a local anesthetic given by injection during surgical procedures and labor and delivery. Chloroprocaine constricts blood vessels resulting in reduced blood loss; this is in contrast to other local anesthetics e.g. lidocaine, which do not do such. Chloroprocaine is an ester anesthetic.
Autotransfusion	Autotransfusion is a process when a person receives their own blood for a transfusion, instead of banked donor blood. Blood can be pre-donated before a surgery, or can be collected during and after the surgery using a device commonly known as the Cell Saver. The Cell Saver is utilized in surgeries where there is expected a large volume blood loss.
Electroconvulsive therapy	Electroconvulsive therapy previously known as electroshock, is a well-established, albeit controversial, psychiatric treatment in which seizures are electrically induced in anesthetized patients for therapeutic effect. Today, ECT is most often used as a treatment for severe major depression which has not responded to other treatment, and is also used in the treatment of mania (often in bipolar disorder), and catatonia. It was first introduced in the 1930s and gained widespread use as a form of treatment in the 1940s and 1950s; today, an estimated 1 million people worldwide receive ECT every year, usually in a course of 6-12 treatments administered 2 or 3 times a week.
Sphygmomanometer	A Sphygmomanometer comprising an inflatable cuff to restrict blood flow, and a mercury or mechanical manometer to measure the pressure. It is always used in conjunction with a means to determine at what pressure blood flow is just starting, and at what pressure it is unimpeded. Manual Sphygmomanometers are used in conjunction with a stethoscope.

Chapter 2. Part II Physiologig Considerations in the PACU

Calcium channel blockers	Calcium channel blockers are a class of drugs and natural substances that disrupt the calcium (Ca^{2+}) conduction of calcium channels.
	The main clinical usage of Calcium channel blockers is to decrease blood pressure. It is for this action that they are used in individuals with hypertension.
Glucocorticoid	Glucocorticoids (GC) are a class of steroid hormones that bind to the Glucocorticoid receptor (GR), which is present in almost every vertebrate animal cell. The name Glucocorticoid derives from their role in the regulation of the metabolism of glucose, their synthesis in the adrenal cortex, and their steroidal structure .
	GCs are part of the feedback mechanism in the immune system that turns immune activity (inflammation) down.
Metabolism	Metabolism is the set of chemical reactions that happen in living organisms to maintain life. These processes allow organisms to grow and reproduce, maintain their structures, and respond to their environments. Metabolism is usually divided into two categories.
Colostomy	A colostomy is a reversible surgical procedure in which a stoma is formed by drawing the healthy end of the large intestine or colon through an incision in the anterior abdominal wall and suturing it into place. This opening, in conjunction with the attached stoma appliance, provides an alternative channel for feces to leave the body.
	Indications
	There are many reasons for this procedure.
Aseptic technique	Aseptic technique refers to a procedure that is performed under sterile conditions. This includes medical and laboratory techniques, such as with microbiological cultures. It includes techniques like flame sterilization.
Latex allergy	Latex allergy is a medical term encompassing a range of allergic reactions to natural rubber latex.

Latex is known to cause 2 of the 4 (or 5) types of hypersensitivity.

The most serious and rare form, type I is an immediate and potentially life-threatening reaction, not unlike the severe reaction some people have to bee stings.

Anesthetic | An anesthetic is a drug that causes anesthesia--reversible loss of sensation. They contrast with analgesics (painkillers), which relieve pain without eliminating sensation. These drugs are generally administered to facilitate surgery.

Chapter 3. Part III Concepts in Anesthetic Agents

Anesthetic	An anesthetic is a drug that causes anesthesia--reversible loss of sensation. They contrast with analgesics (painkillers), which relieve pain without eliminating sensation. These drugs are generally administered to facilitate surgery.
Sedation	Sedation is the reduction of irritability or agitation by administration of sedative drugs, generally to facilitate a medical procedure or diagnostic procedure. Drugs which can be used for sedation include propofol, etomidate, ketamine, fentanyl, and midazolam. Uses Sedation is now typically used in procedures such as endoscopy, vasectomy, RSI (Rapid Sequence Intubation), or minor surgery and in dentistry for reconstructive surgery, some cosmetic surgeries, removal of wisdom teeth, or for high-anxiety patients.
Anesthesia	Anesthesia, traditionally meant the condition of having sensation (including the feeling of pain) blocked or temporarily taken away. It is a pharmacologically induced and reversible state of amnesia, analgesia, loss of responsiveness, loss of skeletal muscle reflexes or decreased stress response, or all simultaneously. This allows patients to undergo surgery and other procedures without the distress and pain they would otherwise experience.
Minimum alveolar concentration	Minimum alveolar concentration is a concept used to compare the strengths, or potency, of anaesthetic vapours; in simple terms, it is defined as the concentration of the vapour in the lungs that is needed to prevent movement (motor response) in 50% of subjects in response to surgical (pain) stimulus. Thus, it is actually a median value; the use of minimum would appear to be descended from the original paper in which the concept appeared, although the term there was minimal alveolar concentration. A lower Minimum alveolar concentration value represents a more potent volatile anesthetic.
Severe acute respiratory syndrome	Severe acute respiratory syndrome is a respiratory disease in humans which is caused by the Severe acute respiratory syndrome coronavirus . There has been one near pandemic to date, between the months of November 2002 and July 2003, with 8,096 known infected cases and 774 deaths (a case-fatality rate of 9.6%) worldwide being listed in the World Health Organization's (WHO) 21 April 2004 concluding report. Within a matter of weeks in early 2003, Severe acute respiratory syndrome spread from the Guangdong province of China to rapidly infect individuals in some 37 countries around the world.

Chapter 3. Part III Concepts in Anesthetic Agents

Hypovolemia	In physiology and medicine, Hypovolemia is a state of decreased blood volume; more specifically, decrease in volume of blood plasma. It is thus the intravascular component of volume contraction (or loss of blood volume due to things such as hemorrhaging or dehydration), but, as it also is the most essential one, Hypovolemia and volume contraction are sometimes used synonymously. It differs from dehydration, which is defined as excessive loss of body water.
Laryngospasm	In medicine, laryngospasm is an uncontrolled/involuntary muscular contraction (spasm) of the laryngeal cords. The condition typically lasts less than 60 seconds, and causes a partial blocking of breathing in, while breathing out remains easier. It may be triggered when the vocal cords or the area of the trachea below the cords detects the entry of water, mucus, blood, or other substance.
Etidocaine	Etidocaine, marketed under the trade name Duranest, is a local anesthetic given by injection during surgical procedures and labor and delivery. Etidocaine has a long duration of activity, and the main disadvantage of using during dentistry is increased bleeding during surgery.
Receptor antagonist	A Receptor antagonist is a type of receptor ligand or drug that does not provoke a biological response itself upon binding to a receptor, but blocks or dampens agonist-mediated responses. In pharmacology, antagonists have affinity but no efficacy for their cognate receptors, and binding will disrupt the interaction and inhibit the function of an agonist or inverse agonist at receptors. Antagonists mediate their effects by binding to the active site or to allosteric sites on receptors, or they may interact at unique binding sites not normally involved in the biological regulation of the receptor's activity.
Cocaine	Cocaine benzoylmethylecgonine (INN) is a crystalline tropane alkaloid that is obtained from the leaves of the coca plant. The name comes from "coca" in addition to the alkaloid suffix -ine, forming cocaine. It is a stimulant of the central nervous system, an appetite suppressant, and a topical anesthetic.
Hypoventilation	In medicine, Hypoventilation occurs when ventilation is inadequate (hypo means 'below') to perform needed gas exchange. By definition it causes an increased concentration of carbon dioxide (hypercapnia) and respiratory acidosis.

It can be caused by medical conditions, such as stroke affecting the brainstem, by holding one's breath, or by drugs, typically when taken in overdose.

Implant

An implant is a medical device manufactured to replace a missing biological structure, support a damaged biological structure, or enhance an existing biological structure. Medical implants are man-made devices, in contrast to a transplant, which is a transplanted biomedical tissue. The surface of implants that contact the body might be made of a biomedical material such as titanium, silicone or apatite depending on what is the most functional.

Transmission

In medicine, transmission is the passing of a disease from an infected individual or group to a previously uninfected individual or group. The microorganisms (bacteria and viruses) that cause disease may be transmitted from one person to another by one or more of the following means:

· droplet contact - coughing or sneezing on another person

· direct physical contact - touching an infected person, including sexual contact

· indirect contact - usually by touching soil contamination or a contaminated surface

· airborne transmission - if the microorganism can remain in the air for long periods

· fecal-oral transmission - usually from contaminated food or water sources

· vector borne transmission - carried by insects or other animals

Microorganisms vary widely in the length of time that they can survive outside the human body, and so vary in how they are transmitted.

Disease can be transmitted in two ways:

· Horizontal disease transmission - from one individual to another in the same generation (peers in the same age group). Horizontal transmission can occur by either direct contact (licking, touching, biting), or indirect contact .

Chapter 3. Part III Concepts in Anesthetic Agents

· Vertical disease transmission - passing a disease causing agent vertically from parent to offspring. Typically the mother transmits the disease by means of bodily fluid, and sometimes breast milk.

Side effect	In medicine, a side effect is an effect, whether therapeutic or adverse, that is secondary to the one intended; although the term is predominantly employed to describe adverse effects, it can also apply to beneficial, but unintended, consequences of the use of a drug.
	Occasionally, drugs are prescribed or procedures performed specifically for their side effects; in that case, said side effect ceases to be a side effect, and is now an intended effect. For instance, X-rays were historically (and are currently) used as an imaging technique; the discovery of their oncolytic capability led to their employ in radiotherapy (ablation of malignant tumours).
Antibacterial	An antibacterial is a compound or substance that kills or slows down the growth of bacteria. The term is often used synonymously with the term antibiotic(s); today, however, with increased knowledge of the causative agents of various infectious diseases, antibiotic(s) has come to denote a broader range of antimicrobial compounds, including anti-fungal and other compounds.
Local anesthetic	A local anesthetic is a drug that causes reversible local anesthesia and a loss of nociception. When it is used on specific nerve pathways (nerve block), effects such as analgesia (loss of pain sensation) and paralysis (loss of muscle power) can be achieved.
	Clinical local anesthetics belong to one of two classes: aminoamide and aminoester local anesthetics.
Intubation	In medicine, Intubation refers to the placement of a tube into an external or internal orifice of the body. Although the term can refer to endoscopic procedures, it is most often used to denote tracheal Intubation. Tracheal Intubation is the placement of a flexible plastic tube into the trachea to protect the patient's airway and provide a means of mechanical ventilation.

35

Chapter 3. Part III Concepts in Anesthetic Agents

Chloroprocaine	Chloroprocaine (often in the hydrochloride salt form as the aforementioned trade names) is a local anesthetic given by injection during surgical procedures and labor and delivery. Chloroprocaine constricts blood vessels resulting in reduced blood loss; this is in contrast to other local anesthetics e.g. lidocaine, which do not do such. Chloroprocaine is an ester anesthetic.
Lidocaine	Lidocaine (Xylocaine) or lignocaine (/ˈlɪgnəˌkeɪn/) (former BAN) is a common local anesthetic and antiarrhythmic drug. Lidocaine is used topically to relieve itching, burning and pain from skin inflammations, injected as a dental anesthetic or as a local anesthetic for minor surgery. History Lidocaine, the first amino amide-type local anesthetic, was first synthesized under the name Xylocaine by Swedish chemist Nils Löfgren in 1943. His colleague Bengt Lundqvist performed the first injection anesthesia experiments on himself.
Prilocaine	Prilocaine is a local anesthetic of the amino amide type. In its injectable form (trade name Citanest), it is often used in dentistry. It is also often combined with lidocaine as a preparation for dermal anesthesia (lidocaine/prilocaine or EMLA), for treatment of conditions like paresthesia.
Bupivacaine	Bupivacaine is a local anaesthetic drug belonging to the amino amide group. AstraZeneca commonly markets it under various trade names, including Marcain, Marcaine, Sensorcaine and Vivacaine. Indications Bupivacaine is indicated for local anaesthesia including infiltration, nerve block, epidural, and intrathecal anaesthesia.
Levobupivacaine	Levobupivacaine is a local anaesthetic drug belonging to the amino amide group. It is the S-enantiomer of bupivacaine.

Levobupivacaine hydrochloride is commonly marketed by AstraZeneca under the trade name Chirocaine.

Mepivacaine

Mepivacaine is a local anesthetic of the amide type. Mepivacaine has a reasonably rapid onset (more rapid than that of procaine) and medium duration of action (shorter than that of procaine) and is marketed under various trade names including Carbocaine and Polocaine.

Mepivacaine became available in the United States in the 1960s.

Ropivacaine

Ropivacaine is a local anaesthetic drug belonging to the amino amide group. The name ropivacaine refers to both the racemate and the marketed S-enantiomer. Ropivacaine hydrochloride is commonly marketed by AstraZeneca under the trade name Naropin.

Tetracaine

Tetracaine is a potent local anesthetic of the ester group. It is mainly used topically in ophthalmology and as an antipruritic, and it has been used in spinal anesthesia.

In biomedical research, tetracaine is used to alter the function of calcium release channels (ryanodine receptors) that control the release of calcium from intracellular stores.

Dermatome

A dermatome is a surgical instrument used to produce thin slices of skin from a donor area, in order to use them for making skin grafts. One of its main applications is for reconstituting skin areas damaged by grade 3 burns or trauma.

Dermatomes can be operated either manually or electrically.

CYam\101

Chapter 3. Part III Concepts in Anesthetic Agents

Postoperative nausea and vomiting	Postoperative nausea and vomiting is an unpleasant complication affecting about a third of the 10% of the population undergoing general anaesthesia each year. This equates to about two million people in the United Kingdom annually. Impact On average the incidence of nausea or vomiting after general anesthesia ranges between 25 and 30% [Cohen 1994].

Chapter 4. Part IV Nursing Care in the PACU

Dead space	In physiology, dead space is air that is inhaled by the body in breathing, but does not take part in gas exchange. Not all the air in each breath is able to be used for the exchange of oxygen and carbon dioxide. About a third of every resting breath is exhaled exactly as it came into the body.
Airway	The pulmonary Airway comprises those parts of the respiratory system through which air flows, conceptually beginning (on inhalation from the external environment) at the nose and mouth, and terminating in the alveoli. It is generally used synonymously with respiratory tract, to avoid sounding overly scientific. From the mouth or nose, inhaled air passes through the pharynx into the trachea, where it separates into the left and right main bronchi at the carina, situated at the level of the second thoracic vertebra.
Anesthesia	Anesthesia, traditionally meant the condition of having sensation (including the feeling of pain) blocked or temporarily taken away. It is a pharmacologically induced and reversible state of amnesia, analgesia, loss of responsiveness, loss of skeletal muscle reflexes or decreased stress response, or all simultaneously. This allows patients to undergo surgery and other procedures without the distress and pain they would otherwise experience.
Auscultation	Auscultation is the technical term for listening to the internal sounds of the body, usually using a stethoscope; based on the Latin verb auscultare 'to listen'. Auscultation is performed for the purposes of examining the circulatory system and respiratory system , as well as the gastrointestinal system (bowel sounds). The term was introduced by René-Théophile-Hyacinthe Laennec.
Palpation	Palpation is used as part of a physical examination in which an object is felt to determine its size, shape, firmness, or location. Palpation should not be confused with palpitation, which is an awareness of the beating of the heart. Palpation is used by various therapists such as medical doctors, practitioners of chiropractic, osteopathic medicine, physical therapists, occupational therapists, and massage therapists, to assess the texture of a patient's tissue (such as swelling or muscle tone), to locate the spatial coordinates of particular anatomical landmarks (e.g., to assess range and quality of joint motion), and assess tenderness through tissue deformation .

Chapter 4. Part IV Nursing Care in the PACU

Pulse oximetry	Pulse oximetry is a non-invasive method allowing the monitoring of the oxygenation of a patient's hemoglobin.
	A sensor is placed on a thin part of the patient's body, usually a fingertip or earlobe, or in the case of a neonate, across a foot, and a light containing both red and infrared wavelengths is passed from one side to the other. Changing absorbance of each of the two wavelengths is measured, allowing determination of the absorbances due to the pulsing arterial blood alone, excluding venous blood, skin, bone, muscle, fat, and (in most cases) fingernail polish.
Capnography	Capnography is the monitoring of the concentration or partial pressure of carbon dioxide (CO_2) in the respiratory gases. Its main development has been as a monitoring tool for use during anaesthesia and intensive care. It is usually presented as a graph of expiratory CO_2 plotted against time, or, less commonly, but more usefully, expired volume.
Pain management	Pain management is a branch of medicine employing an interdisciplinary approach for easing the suffering and improving the quality of life of those living with pain. The typical pain management team includes medical practitioners, clinical psychologists, physiotherapists, occupational therapists, and nurse practitioners. Pain sometimes resolves promptly once the underlying trauma or pathology has healed, and is treated by one practitioner, with drugs such as analgesics and (occasionally) anxiolytics.
Patient education	Patient education is the process by which health professionals and others impart information to patients that will alter their health behaviors or improve their health status. Education providers may include: physicians, registered dietitians, nurses, hospital discharge planners, medical social workers, psychologists, disease or disability advocacy groups, special interest groups, and pharmaceutical companies.
Hypoventilation	In medicine, Hypoventilation occurs when ventilation is inadequate (hypo means 'below') to perform needed gas exchange. By definition it causes an increased concentration of carbon dioxide (hypercapnia) and respiratory acidosis.
	It can be caused by medical conditions, such as stroke affecting the brainstem, by holding one's breath, or by drugs, typically when taken in overdose.

Chapter 4. Part IV Nursing Care in the PACU

Laryngospasm	In medicine, laryngospasm is an uncontrolled/involuntary muscular contraction (spasm) of the laryngeal cords. The condition typically lasts less than 60 seconds, and causes a partial blocking of breathing in, while breathing out remains easier. It may be triggered when the vocal cords or the area of the trachea below the cords detects the entry of water, mucus, blood, or other substance.
Airway obstruction	Airway obstruction is a respiratory problem caused by increased resistance in the bronchioles (usually from a decreased radius of the bronchioles) that reduces the amount of air inhaled in each breath and the oxygen that reaches the pulmonary arteries. It is different from airway restriction . Obstruction can be measured using spirometry.
Pulmonary edema	Pulmonary edema is fluid accumulation in the lungs. It leads to impaired gas exchange and may cause respiratory failure. It is due to either failure of the heart to remove fluid from the lung circulation or a direct injury to the lung parenchyma .
Cricothyrotomy	A cricothyrotomy is an incision made through the skin and cricothyroid membrane to establish a patent airway during certain life-threatening situations, such as airway obstruction by a foreign body, angioedema, or massive facial trauma. Cricothyrotomy is nearly always performed as a last resort in cases where orotracheal and nasotracheal intubation are impossible or contraindicated. Cricothyrotomy is easier and quicker to perform than tracheotomy, does not require manipulation of the cervical spine, and is associated with fewer complications.
Laryngoscopy	Laryngoscopy is a medical procedure that is used to obtain a view of the vocal folds and the glottis. Laryngoscopy may be performed to facilitate tracheal intubation during general anesthesia or cardiopulmonary resuscitation or for procedures on the larynx or other parts of the upper tracheobronchial tree. Direct laryngoscopy is carried out (usually) with the patient lying on his or her back; the laryngoscope is inserted into the mouth on the right side and flipped to the left to trap and move the tongue out of the line of sight, and, depending on the type of blade used, inserted either anterior or posterior to the epiglottis and then lifted with an upwards and forward motion ("away from you and towards the roof ").

Oropharynx	The Oropharynx reaches from the Uvula to the level of the hyoid bone.

It opens anteriorly, through the isthmus faucium, into the mouth, while in its lateral wall, between the two palatine arches, is the palatine tonsil.

Although older resources have stated that Fusobacterium is a common occurrence in the human Oropharynx, the current consensus is that Fusobacterium should always be treated as a pathogen.

The name is formed from their initials:

· Haemophilus

· Actinobacillus actinomycetemcomitans

· Cardiobacterium hominis

· Eikenella corrodens

· Kingella

All of these organisms are part of the normal oropharyngeal flora which grow slowly, prefer a carbon dioxide-enriched atmosphere and share an enhanced capacity to produce endocardial infections, especially in young children. |
| Intubation | In medicine, Intubation refers to the placement of a tube into an external or internal orifice of the body. Although the term can refer to endoscopic procedures, it is most often used to denote tracheal Intubation. Tracheal Intubation is the placement of a flexible plastic tube into the trachea to protect the patient's airway and provide a means of mechanical ventilation. |

Chapter 4. Part IV Nursing Care in the PACU

Endotracheal tube	An Endotracheal tube is used in general anaesthesia, intensive care and emergency medicine for airway management, mechanical ventilation and as an alternative route for many drugs if an IV line cannot be established. The tube is inserted into a patient's trachea in order to ensure that the airway is not closed off and that air is able to reach the lungs. The Endotracheal tube is regarded as the most reliable available method for protecting a patient's airway.
Laryngoscope	A Laryngoscope is a medical device that is used to obtain a view of the vocal folds and the glottis, which is the space between the cords. The first Laryngoscope was invented in 1854 by Manuel Patricio Rodríguez García.
Tracheal Intubation	Tracheal intubation, usually simply referred to as intubation, is the placement of a flexible plastic tube into the trachea (windpipe) to maintain an open airway or to serve as a conduit through which to administer certain drugs. It is frequently performed in critically injured, ill or anesthetized patients to facilitate ventilation of the lungs, including mechanical ventilation, and to prevent the possibility of asphyxiation or airway obstruction. The most widely used route is orotracheal, in which an endotracheal tube is passed through the mouth and vocal apparatus into the trachea.
Side effect	In medicine, a side effect is an effect, whether therapeutic or adverse, that is secondary to the one intended; although the term is predominantly employed to describe adverse effects, it can also apply to beneficial, but unintended, consequences of the use of a drug. Occasionally, drugs are prescribed or procedures performed specifically for their side effects; in that case, said side effect ceases to be a side effect, and is now an intended effect. For instance, X-rays were historically (and are currently) used as an imaging technique; the discovery of their oncolytic capability led to their employ in radiotherapy (ablation of malignant tumours).
Cocaine	Cocaine benzoylmethylecgonine (INN) is a crystalline tropane alkaloid that is obtained from the leaves of the coca plant. The name comes from "coca" in addition to the alkaloid suffix -ine, forming cocaine. It is a stimulant of the central nervous system, an appetite suppressant, and a topical anesthetic.
Cochlear implant	A cochlear implant is a surgically implanted electronic device that provides a sense of sound to a person who is profoundly deaf or severely hard of hearing. The cochlear implant is often referred to as a bionic ear.

As of April 2009, approximately 188,000 people worldwide had received cochlear implants; in the United States, about 30,000 adults and over 30,000 children are recipients.

Myringotomy	Myringotomy is a surgical procedure in which a tiny incision is created in the eardrum, so as to relieve pressure caused by the excessive build-up of fluid, or to drain pus. Myringotomy is often performed as a treatment for otitis media. If a patient requires myringotomy for drainage or ventilation of the middle ear, this generally implies that the Eustachian tube is either partially or completely obstructed and is not able to perform this function in its usual physiologic fashion.
Stapedectomy	A stapedectomy is a surgical procedure of the middle ear performed to improve hearing. The world's first stapedectomy is credited to Dr. John J. Shea, Jr., performed in May, 1956, on a 54-year-old housewife who could no longer hear even with a hearing aid. In recent years, Dr. William H. Lippy has been credited with major advances for the surgical procedure and is well known for several thousand stapedectomy revision surgeries he has performed.
Stent	In medicine, a stent is an artificial 'tube' inserted into a natural passage/conduit in the body to prevent, or counteract, a disease-induced, localized flow constriction. The term may also refer to a tube used to temporarily hold such a natural conduit open to allow access for surgery.
	Etymology
	The origin of the word stent remains unsettled.
Laryngeal mask airway	The laryngeal mask airway is a supraglottic airway device invented by Archie Brain, a British anaesthetist.
	Description
	Laryngeal masks consist of a tube with an inflatable cuff that is inserted into the pharynx. They cause less pain and coughing than an endotracheal tube, and are much easier to insert.

Chapter 4. Part IV Nursing Care in the PACU

Dacryocystorhinostomy	Dacryocystorhinostomy is a surgical procedure to restore the flow of tears into the nose from the lacrimal sac when the nasolacrimal duct does not function.
	Process
	Traditional
	A small incision is made on the side of the nose and some bone is removed to make a connection to the nose. Drains are left behind to prevent the gap from closing and are removed after a few months.
Dermatochalasis	Dermatochalasis is a medical condition. It is defined as an excess of skin in the upper or lower eyelid. It may be either an acquired or a congenital condition. It is generally treated with blepharoplasty.
Enucleation	As a general surgical technique, enucleation refers to the surgical removal of a mass without cutting into or dissecting it.
	Removal of the eye
	Enucleation refers to removal of the eyeball itself, while leaving surrounding tissues intact.
	Removal of oral cysts and tumors
	In the context of oral pathology, enucleation involves removal of all tissue (both hard and soft) involved in a lesion.
Hydroxylapatite	Hydroxylapatite, is a naturally occurring mineral form of calcium apatite with the formula $Ca_5(PO_4)_3(OH)$, but is usually written $Ca_{10}(PO_4)_6(OH)_2$ to denote that the crystal unit cell comprises two entities. Hydroxylapatite is the hydroxyl endmember of the complex apatite group. The OH^- ion can be replaced by fluoride, chloride or carbonate, producing fluorapatite or chlorapatite.

Chapter 4. Part IV Nursing Care in the PACU

Ptosis	Ptosis is a (drooping) of the upper or lower eyelid. The drooping may be worse after being awake longer, when the individual's muscles are tired. This condition is sometimes called "lazy eye", but that term normally refers to amblyopia.
Minimum alveolar concentration	Minimum alveolar concentration is a concept used to compare the strengths, or potency, of anaesthetic vapours; in simple terms, it is defined as the concentration of the vapour in the lungs that is needed to prevent movement (motor response) in 50% of subjects in response to surgical (pain) stimulus. Thus, it is actually a median value; the use of minimum would appear to be descended from the original paper in which the concept appeared, although the term there was minimal alveolar concentration. A lower Minimum alveolar concentration value represents a more potent volatile anesthetic.
Mediastinoscopy	Mediastinoscopy is a procedure that enables visualization of the contents of the mediastinum, usually for the purpose of obtaining a biopsy. Mediastinoscopy is often used for staging of lymph nodes of lung cancer or for diagnosing other conditions affecting structures in the mediastinum such as sarcoidosis or lymphoma. Mediastinoscopy involves making an incision approximately 1 cm above the suprasternal notch of the sternum, or breast bone.
Segmental resection	Segmental resection is a surgical procedure to remove part of an organ or gland. It may also be used to remove a tumor and normal tissue around it. In lung cancer surgery, segmental **resection refers to removing a section of a lobe of the lung.**
Reduction	Reduction is a medical procedure to restore a fracture or dislocation to the correct alignment. When a bone fractures, the fragments lose their alignment in the form of displacement or angulation. For the fractured bone to heal without any deformity the bony fragments must be re-aligned to their normal anatomical position.
Commissurotomy	A commissurotomy is a surgical incision of a commissure in the body, as one made in the heart at the edges of the commissure formed by cardiac valves, or one made in the brain to treat certain psychiatric disorders.

Patients with scleroderma, a disease that thickens and hardens the skin, sometimes require oral commissurotomy to open the corners of the mouth, the commissures, to allow dental treatment. This procedure often leaves characteristic scars.

Pericardiectomy	Pericardiectomy is the surgical removal of part or most of the pericardium. This operation is most commonly done to relieve constrictive pericarditis, or to remove a pericardium that is calcified and fibrous. There are many etiologies for constrictive pericarditis and it is better to know the exact cause as the post operative morbidity, mortality and life expectancy are strongly influenced by the cause.
Anesthetic	An anesthetic is a drug that causes anesthesia--reversible loss of sensation. They contrast with analgesics (painkillers), which relieve pain without eliminating sensation. These drugs are generally administered to facilitate surgery.
Arthroscopy	Arthroscopy is a minimally invasive surgical procedure in which an examination and sometimes treatment of damage of the interior of a joint is performed using an arthroscope, a type of endoscope that is inserted into the joint through a small incision. Arthroscopic procedures can be performed either to evaluate or to treat many orthopedic conditions including torn floating cartilage, torn surface cartilage, ACL reconstruction, and trimming damaged cartilage. The advantage of arthroscopy over traditional open surgery is that the joint does not have to be opened up fully.
Fasciotomy	Fasciotomy is cut to relieve tension or pressure (and treat the resulting loss of circulation to an area of tissue or muscle). Fasciotomy is a limb-saving procedure when used to treat acute compartment syndrome. It is also sometimes used to treat chronic compartment stress syndrome.
Harrington rod	The Harrington implant (or Harrington rod) is a stainless steel surgical device. Historically, this rod was implanted along the spinal column to treat, among other conditions, a lateral or coronal-plane curvature of the spine, or scoliosis. Up to one million people had Harrington rods implanted for scoliosis between the early 1960s and the late 1990s.

Chapter 4. Part IV Nursing Care in the PACU

Osteotomy	An osteotomy is a surgical operation whereby a bone is cut to shorten, lengthen, or change its alignment. It is sometimes performed to correct a hallux valgus, or to straighten a bone that has healed crookedly following a fracture. It is also used to correct a coxa vara, genu valgum, and genu varum.
Joint replacement	A joint replacement is needed when "an arthritic or damaged joint is removed and replaced with an artificial joint, called a prosthesis". Arthroplasty [from Greek arthron, joint, limb, articulate, + -plassein, to form, mould, forge, feign, make an image of], or joint replacement surgery, is a procedure of orthopedic surgery, in which the arthritic or dysfunctional joint surface is replaced with an orthopaedic prosthesis. When joint replacement surgery occurs, the artificial surfaces of the joint replacement are shaped in such a way as to allow joint movement similar to that of a healthy and natural joint.
Autotransfusion	Autotransfusion is a process when a person receives their own blood for a transfusion, instead of banked donor blood. Blood can be pre-donated before a surgery, or can be collected during and after the surgery using a device commonly known as the Cell Saver. The Cell Saver is utilized in surgeries where there is expected a large volume blood loss.
Hand surgery	The field of hand surgery deals with both surgical and non-surgical treatment of conditions and problems that may take place in the hand or upper extremity (commonly from the tip of the hand to the shoulder). Hand surgery may be practiced by graduates of general surgery, orthopedic surgery and plastic surgery. Plastic surgeons and orthopedic surgeons receive significant training in hand surgery during their residency training, with some graduates continuing on to do an additional one year hand fellowship.
Recurrent laryngeal nerve	The Recurrent laryngeal nerve is a branch of the vagus nerve (tenth cranial nerve) that supplies motor function and sensation to the larynx (voice box). It travels within the endoneurial sheath. It is the nerve of the 6th Branchial Arch.
Colostomy	A colostomy is a reversible surgical procedure in which a stoma is formed by drawing the healthy end of the large intestine or colon through an incision in the anterior abdominal wall and suturing it into place. This opening, in conjunction with the attached stoma appliance, provides an alternative channel for feces to leave the body. Indications There are many reasons for this procedure.

Chapter 4. Part IV Nursing Care in the PACU

Intussusception	An intussusception is a medical condition in which a part of the intestine has invaginated into another section of intestine, similar to the way in which the parts of a collapsible telescope slide into one another. This can often result in an obstruction. The part that prolapses into the other is called the intussusceptum, and the part that receives it is called the intussuscipiens.
Pyloromyotomy	Pyloromyotomy is a surgical procedure in which an incision is made in the longitudinal and circular muscles of the pylorus. It is used to treat hypertrophic pyloric stenosis.It is also known as Ramstedt,s Operation.
Angioplasty	Angioplasty is the technique of mechanically widening a narrowed or obstructed blood vessel, typically as a result of atherosclerosis. An empty and collapsed balloon on a guide wire, known as a balloon catheter, is passed into the narrowed locations and then inflated to a fixed size using water pressures some 75 to 500 times normal blood pressure (6 to 20 atmospheres). The balloon crushes the fatty deposits, opening up the blood vessel for improved flow, and the balloon is then collapsed and withdrawn.
Orchiopexy	Orchiopexy is a surgery to move an undescended testicle into the scrotum and permanently fix it there. It is performed by a pediatric urologist or surgeon on boys with cryptorchidism, typically before they reach the age of two. Some patients remain undiagnosed until their teenage years and undergo the surgery at that time.
Pyeloplasty	Pyeloplasty is the surgical reconstruction or revision of the renal pelvis to drain and decompress the kidney. Most commonly it is performed to treat an uretero-pelvic junction obstruction if residual renal function is adequate.

This revision of the renal pelvis treats the obstruction by excising the stenotic area of the renal pelvis or uretero-pelvic junction and creating a more capacious conduit using the tissue of the remaining ureter and renal pelvis. |
| Spermatocelectomy | A spermatocelectomy is a surgical procedure performed to separate the epididymis from the spermatocele. The patient is given an anesthetic in the groin and a small incision is made into the scrotum. The surgeon pulls the testicle and epididymis to the incision and separates the spermatocele by tying it off with a suture. |

Clam101

Kidney transplantation	Kidney transplantation is the organ transplant of a kidney into a patient with end-stage renal disease. Kidney transplantation is typically classified as deceased-donor (formerly known as cadaveric) or living-donor transplantation depending on the source of the donor organ. Living-donor renal transplants are further characterized as genetically related (living-related) or non-related (living-unrelated) transplants, depending on whether a biological relationship exists between the donor and recipient.
Percutaneous nephrolithotomy	Percutaneous nephrolithotomy is a surgical procedure to remove stones from the kidney by a small puncture wound (up to about 1 cm) through the skin. It is most suitable to remove stones of more than 2 cm in size. It is usually done under general anesthesia or spinal anesthesia.
Colporrhaphy	Colporrhaphy is a surgical procedure in humans that repairs a defect in the wall of the vagina. It is the surgical intervention for both cystocele (protrusion of the urinary bladder into the vagina) and rectocele (protrusion of the rectum into the vagina). The repair may be to either or both of the anterior (front) or posterior (rear) vaginal walls, thus the origin of some of its alternative names.
Colpocleisis	Colpocleisis is a procedure involving closure of the vagina. It is used to treat vaginal prolapse.
Mastopexy	Mastopexy surgery denotes a group of elective surgical procedures designed either to lift or to change the shape of a woman's breasts. Besides lifting the breast tissue and removing skin, a mastopexy might also include repositioning the areola and the nipple. In practice, a mastopexy can be effected as a discrete surgery, or as a subordinate surgery comprehended within a breast augmentation done for the emplacement of breast implants.
Breast reduction	Breast reduction is a common surgical procedure which involves the reduction in the size of breasts by excising fat, skin, breast implants and glandular tissue; it may also involve a procedure to counteract drooping of the breasts. As with breast augmentation, this procedure is typically performed on women, but may also be performed on men afflicted by gynecomastia. In 2005, over 113,000 women had breast reductions, an increase of 11 percent from 2004.

Chapter 4. Part IV Nursing Care in the PACU

Abdominoplasty	Abdominoplasty is a cosmetic surgery procedure used to make the abdomen more firm. The surgery involves the removal of excess skin and fat from the middle and lower abdomen in order to tighten the muscle and fascia of the abdominal wall. This type of surgery is usually sought by patients with loose tissues after pregnancy or individuals with sagging after major weight loss.
Dermabrasion	Dermabrasion is a surgical procedure that involves the controlled abrasion (wearing away) of the upper layers of the skin with sandpaper or other mechanical means. Nowadays it has become common to use CO_2 or Erbium:YAG laser as well. The procedure requires a local anaesthetic.
Otoplasty	Otoplasty, is a cosmetic surgery to change the appearance of a person's external ears. Otoplasty can take many forms, such as bringing the ears closer to the head (often called ear pinning), reducing the size of very big ears, or reshaping various bends in the cartilage. Other reconstructive procedures deal with the deformed, or absent (microtic) ears.
Local anesthetic	A local anesthetic is a drug that causes reversible local anesthesia and a loss of nociception. When it is used on specific nerve pathways (nerve block), effects such as analgesia (loss of pain sensation) and paralysis (loss of muscle power) can be achieved.
	Clinical local anesthetics belong to one of two classes: aminoamide and aminoester local anesthetics.
Rhytidectomy	A facelift, technically known as a rhytidectomy is a type of cosmetic surgery procedure used to give a more youthful appearance. It usually involves the removal of excess facial skin, with or without the tightening of underlying tissues, and the redraping of the skin on the patient's face and neck. The first facelift was performed in Berlin in 1901 by Eugen Holländer.
Tissue expansion	Tissue expansion is a technique used by plastic and restorative surgeons to cause the body to grow additional skin, bone or other tissues.
	Skin expansion

Keeping living tissues under tension causes new cells to form and the amount of tissue to increase. In some cases, this may be accomplished by the implantation of inflatable balloons under the skin .

Free flap	The terms free flap and free tissue transfer are synonymous labels used to describe the movement of tissue from one site on the body to another. "Free" implies that the tissue, along with its blood supply, is detached from the original location ("donor site") and then transferred to another location ("recipient site"). This is in contrast to a "pedicled" flap in which tissue is left attached to the donor site and simply transposed to a new location keeping the "pedicle" intact as a conduit to supply the tissue with blood.
Cleft lip and palate	Cleft lip (cheiloschisis) and cleft palate (palatoschisis), which can also occur together as cleft lip and palate, are variations of a type of clefting congenital deformity caused by abnormal facial development during gestation. A cleft is a fissure or opening--a gap. It is the non-fusion of the body's natural structures that form before birth.
Liposuction	Liposuction, liposculpture suction lipectomy or simply lipo ("suction-assisted fat removal") is a cosmetic surgery operation that removes fat from many different sites on the human body. Areas affected can range from the abdomen, thighs and buttocks, to the neck, backs of the arms and elsewhere.
	Several factors limit the amount of fat that can be safely removed in one session.
Transmission	In medicine, transmission is the passing of a disease from an infected individual or group to a previously uninfected individual or group. The microorganisms (bacteria and viruses) that cause disease may be transmitted from one person to another by one or more of the following means:

· droplet contact - coughing or sneezing on another person

· direct physical contact - touching an infected person, including sexual contact

· indirect contact - usually by touching soil contamination or a contaminated surface

· airborne transmission - if the microorganism can remain in the air for long periods

· fecal-oral transmission - usually from contaminated food or water sources

· vector borne transmission - carried by insects or other animals

Microorganisms vary widely in the length of time that they can survive outside the human body, and so vary in how they are transmitted.

Disease can be transmitted in two ways:

· Horizontal disease transmission - from one individual to another in the same generation (peers in the same age group). Horizontal transmission can occur by either direct contact (licking, touching, biting), or indirect contact .

· Vertical disease transmission - passing a disease causing agent vertically from parent to offspring. Typically the mother transmits the disease by means of bodily fluid, and sometimes breast milk.

Poliomyelitis	Poliomyelitis is an acute viral infectious disease spread from person to person, primarily via the fecal-oral route. Although around 90% of polio infections cause no symptoms at all, affected individuals can exhibit a range of symptoms if the virus enters the blood stream. In about 1% of cases the virus enters the central nervous system, preferentially infecting and destroying motor neurons, leading to muscle weakness and acute flaccid paralysis. Different types of paralysis may occur, depending on the nerves involved. Spinal polio is the most common form, characterized by asymmetric paralysis that most often involves the legs. Bulbar polio leads to weakness of muscles innervated by cranial nerves. Bulbospinal polio is a combination of bulbar and spinal paralysis.

Chapter 5. Part V Special Considerations

Hypovolemia	In physiology and medicine, Hypovolemia is a state of decreased blood volume; more specifically, decrease in volume of blood plasma. It is thus the intravascular component of volume contraction (or loss of blood volume due to things such as hemorrhaging or dehydration), but, as it also is the most essential one, Hypovolemia and volume contraction are sometimes used synonymously.
	It differs from dehydration, which is defined as excessive loss of body water.
Local anesthetic	A local anesthetic is a drug that causes reversible local anesthesia and a loss of nociception. When it is used on specific nerve pathways (nerve block), effects such as analgesia (loss of pain sensation) and paralysis (loss of muscle power) can be achieved.
	Clinical local anesthetics belong to one of two classes: aminoamide and aminoester local anesthetics.
Ptosis	Ptosis is a (drooping) of the upper or lower eyelid. The drooping may be worse after being awake longer, when the individual's muscles are tired. This condition is sometimes called "lazy eye", but that term normally refers to amblyopia.
Carboxyhemoglobin	Carboxyhemoglobin is a stable complex of carbon monoxide and hemoglobin that forms in red blood cells when carbon monoxide is inhaled or produced in normal metabolism. Large quantities of it hinder delivery of oxygen to the body. Tobacco smoking (through carbon monoxide inhalation) raises the blood levels of COHb by a factor of several times from its normal concentrations.
Airway	The pulmonary Airway comprises those parts of the respiratory system through which air flows, conceptually beginning (on inhalation from the external environment) at the nose and mouth, and terminating in the alveoli. It is generally used synonymously with respiratory tract, to avoid sounding overly scientific.
	From the mouth or nose, inhaled air passes through the pharynx into the trachea, where it separates into the left and right main bronchi at the carina, situated at the level of the second thoracic vertebra.

Chapter 5. Part V Special Considerations

Hypoventilation	In medicine, Hypoventilation occurs when ventilation is inadequate (hypo means 'below') to perform needed gas exchange. By definition it causes an increased concentration of carbon dioxide (hypercapnia) and respiratory acidosis.
	It can be caused by medical conditions, such as stroke affecting the brainstem, by holding one's breath, or by drugs, typically when taken in overdose.
Anesthesia	Anesthesia, traditionally meant the condition of having sensation (including the feeling of pain) blocked or temporarily taken away. It is a pharmacologically induced and reversible state of amnesia, analgesia, loss of responsiveness, loss of skeletal muscle reflexes or decreased stress response, or all simultaneously. This allows patients to undergo surgery and other procedures without the distress and pain they would otherwise experience.
Articaine	Articaine is a dental local anesthetic. It is the most widely used local anesthetic in a number of European countries and is available in many countries around the world. History This drug was first synthesized by Rusching in 1969, and brought to the market in Germany by Hoechst AG, a life-sciences German company, under the brand name Ultracain.
Anesthetic	An anesthetic is a drug that causes anesthesia--reversible loss of sensation. They contrast with analgesics (painkillers), which relieve pain without eliminating sensation. These drugs are generally administered to facilitate surgery.
Barotrauma	Barotrauma is physical damage to body tissues caused by a difference in pressure between an air space inside or beside the body and the surrounding fluid. Barotrauma typically occurs to air spaces within a body when that body moves to or from a higher pressure environment, such as when a SCUBA diver, a free-diving diver or an airplane passenger ascends or descends, or during uncontrolled decompression of a pressure vessel. Boyle's law defines the relationship between the volume of the air space and the ambient pressure.

Chapter 5. Part V Special Considerations

Intubation	In medicine, Intubation refers to the placement of a tube into an external or internal orifice of the body. Although the term can refer to endoscopic procedures, it is most often used to denote tracheal Intubation. Tracheal Intubation is the placement of a flexible plastic tube into the trachea to protect the patient's airway and provide a means of mechanical ventilation.
Laryngospasm	In medicine, laryngospasm is an uncontrolled/involuntary muscular contraction (spasm) of the laryngeal cords. The condition typically lasts less than 60 seconds, and causes a partial blocking of breathing in, while breathing out remains easier. It may be triggered when the vocal cords or the area of the trachea below the cords detects the entry of water, mucus, blood, or other substance.
Dead space	In physiology, dead space is air that is inhaled by the body in breathing, but does not take part in gas exchange. Not all the air in each breath is able to be used for the exchange of oxygen and carbon dioxide. About a third of every resting breath is exhaled exactly as it came into the body.
Aseptic technique	Aseptic technique refers to a procedure that is performed under sterile conditions. This includes medical and laboratory techniques, such as with microbiological cultures. It includes techniques like flame sterilization.
Severe acute respiratory syndrome	Severe acute respiratory syndrome is a respiratory disease in humans which is caused by the Severe acute respiratory syndrome coronavirus . There has been one near pandemic to date, between the months of November 2002 and July 2003, with 8,096 known infected cases and 774 deaths (a case-fatality rate of 9.6%) worldwide being listed in the World Health Organization's (WHO) 21 April 2004 concluding report. Within a matter of weeks in early 2003, Severe acute respiratory syndrome spread from the Guangdong province of China to rapidly infect individuals in some 37 countries around the world.
Pain management	Pain management is a branch of medicine employing an interdisciplinary approach for easing the suffering and improving the quality of life of those living with pain. The typical pain management team includes medical practitioners, clinical psychologists, physiotherapists, occupational therapists, and nurse practitioners. Pain sometimes resolves promptly once the underlying trauma or pathology has healed, and is treated by one practitioner, with drugs such as analgesics and (occasionally) anxiolytics.
Airway obstruction	Airway obstruction is a respiratory problem caused by increased resistance in the bronchioles (usually from a decreased radius of the bronchioles) that reduces the amount of air inhaled in each breath and the oxygen that reaches the pulmonary arteries. It is different from airway restriction .

Go to **Cram101.com** for Interactive Practice Exams for this book or virtually any of your books.
And, **NEVER** highlight a book again!

Chapter 5. Part V Special Considerations

	Obstruction can be measured using spirometry.
Laryngoscopy	Laryngoscopy is a medical procedure that is used to obtain a view of the vocal folds and the glottis. Laryngoscopy may be performed to facilitate tracheal intubation during general anesthesia or cardiopulmonary resuscitation or for procedures on the larynx or other parts of the upper tracheobronchial tree.
	Direct laryngoscopy is carried out (usually) with the patient lying on his or her back; the laryngoscope is inserted into the mouth on the right side and flipped to the left to trap and move the tongue out of the line of sight, and, depending on the type of blade used, inserted either anterior or posterior to the epiglottis and then lifted with an upwards and forward motion ("away from you and towards the roof ").
Antibacterial	An antibacterial is a compound or substance that kills or slows down the growth of bacteria. The term is often used synonymously with the term antibiotic(s); today, however, with increased knowledge of the causative agents of various infectious diseases, antibiotic(s) has come to denote a broader range of antimicrobial compounds, including anti-fungal and other compounds.
Cocaine	Cocaine benzoylmethylecgonine (INN) is a crystalline tropane alkaloid that is obtained from the leaves of the coca plant. The name comes from "coca" in addition to the alkaloid suffix -ine, forming cocaine. It is a stimulant of the central nervous system, an appetite suppressant, and a topical anesthetic.
Convection	Convection is the movement of molecules within fluids (i.e. liquids, gases and rheids). It cannot take place in solids, since neither bulk current flows or significant diffusion can take place in solids.
	Convection is one of the major modes of heat transfer and mass transfer.
Bacteriostatic agent	Bacteriostatic antibiotics limit the growth of bacteria by interfering with bacterial protein production, DNA replication, or other aspects of bacterial cellular metabolism.

Bacteriostatic antibiotics inhibit growth and reproduction of bacteria without killing them; killing is done by bactericidal agents. Bacteriostatic agents must work with the immune system to remove the microorganisms from the body. However, there is not always a precise distinction between them and bactericides; high concentrations of some bacteriostatic agents are also bactericidal, whereas low concentrations of some bacteriocidal agents are bacteriostatic.

Infection control	Infection control is the discipline concerned with preventing nosocomial or healthcare-associated infection. As such, it is a practical (rather than an academic) sub-discipline of epidemiology. It is an essential (though often under-recognized and under-supported) part of the infrastructure of health care.
Cardiogenic shock	Cardiogenic shock is based upon an inadequate circulation of blood due to primary failure of the ventricles of the heart to function effectively. Since this is a type of shock there is insufficient perfusion of tissue (i.e. the heart) to meet the required demands for oxygen and nutrients. This leads to cell death from oxygen starvation (hypoxia) and nutrient starvation (eg hypoglycemia).
Neurogenic shock	Neurogenic shock is shock caused by the sudden loss of the autonomic nervous system signals to the smooth muscle in vessel walls. This can result from severe central nervous system (brain and spinal cord) damage. With the sudden loss of background sympathetic stimulation, the vessels suddenly relax resulting in a sudden decrease in peripheral vascular resistance (vasodilation) and decreased blood pressure.